Table of Contents

Incorporating High-Intensity Interval Training (HIIT) into Your Fitness Routine

An In-Depth Guide to 6 Best HIIT Exercises - With and Without Equipment

1. Introduction to HIIT (High-Intensity Interval Training)

EXPERT TIP! Everyone has a unique fitness benchmark and physiology, so train accordingly and at the intensity best suited. While HIIT has shown to provide many benefits, overdoing it and not recovering can lead to decreased performance. Balance is key. To work on this, see a certified trainer before tweaking your fitness regimen.

The body benefits from HIIT in a myriad of ways. It can help you torch calories, which may then make it easier to achieve a calorie deficit and lose body fat, as well as provide a change from the traditional moderate-pace cardio and muscle-toning workouts to complement your overall fitness routine. HIIT can also cause a longer period of excess post-exercise oxygen consumption (EPOC) and significant changes in your metabolic rate, meaning you'll continue burning more calories after each session is over. HIIT can have additional benefits over steady-state cardio. High-intensity intervals can increase your heart rate, maximize your oxygen consumption, and increase your afterburn, i.e., the number of calories burned after exercise, thus increasing the resting metabolic rate (RMR) which means you'll continue to burn calories. Plus, the quick brief high-intensity moments might feel like you're not working out for very long, which makes it more engaging for some people than if they were doing moderate-intensity cardio for a longer time.

High-intensity interval training, or HIIT, has been garnering a lot of attention in the fitness world when it comes to weight loss. But, what is it? HIIT sessions combine short bursts of intense exercise with periods of rest, like an activity that sends your heart rate soaring for about 10 minutes. These periods of going all-out are followed by active recovery or complete rest, during which your heart rate comes down slightly so that you can go full-force for the next sprint. The exact work-to-rest ratio varies, and the goals may change (e.g., to build strength versus endurance), but usually, you work as hard as you can for a short interval, rest just enough to recover, then repeat for multiple intervals or rounds. You can also experiment with low-, moderate-, and high-intensity intervals, the first for warm-up, the second for work, and the last for the hard effort or various HIIT schemes like Tabata, fartlek, and more.

2. Benefits of HIIT Workouts

One of the most common tactics for losing fat is through HIIT (high-intensity interval training). It's claimed to be really effective when it comes to burning calories and building muscle. If you do it right, HIIT involves a lot of big movements. The exercises make use of huge muscle groups, and you can use a lot of energy with a six-pack. Because research shows that you are able to burn more calories after an intense workout than you normally would. That's a process called EPOC (excess post-exercise oxygen consumption). It's a significant advantage as it can help you absorb more oxygen after heavy exercise. It can also help you recover by increasing your heart rate and revealing internal processes. Thus, it increases metabolism and helps those who are focused on burning calories.

High-Intensity Interval Training, abbreviated as HIIT, is a workout that improves heart metabolism, blood pressure, and cardiovascular fitness. It also aids in weight loss by reducing abdominal fat and increasing muscle strength. HIIT workouts, which can be done with or without equipment, are also less time-consuming while providing the same benefits in comparison to long sessions in the gym. Using HIIT, you can strengthen your glutes and quadriceps by 37 percent and be active throughout the day. The workout can also be specifically designed to meet gender and age-specific needs. HIIT workouts produce better results in males, but they are also good for females as they burn more sugar than fat in their bodies.

3. Key Principles of HIIT

Two key principles of HIIT are work-rest ratios and intensity. The work-to-rest ratio in a HIIT workout is typically 2:1 to 1:5. The work interval, or 'ON' time, can be anything between five seconds to eight minutes, although the actual time can be manipulated to a certain degree based on the intensity that the work is being performed at. The rest interval, or 'OFF' time, is typically a passive recovery where you sit around and/or do nothing before you begin your next work interval, although it needs to be at a light intensity too. Note that work-to-rest ratios can change quite a bit based on your specific training goals and are not set in stone.

HIIT workouts use a few key principles, such as work-rest ratios, that are very easy to manipulate in a gym environment. They are easily adaptable and can produce a wide range of physiological benefits, which can be important for training different energy systems for various sports and activities. HIIT includes all sorts of different interval training. Specifically, work-to-rest ratios and intensity levels can be manipulated, and the exercise mode can be whatever you want it to be. But, for the purpose of this article, I will offer you some different movements and exercises you could use in your HIIT workouts, both with and without a resistance or strength-building component.

High-intensity interval training (HIIT) is an effective way to get a lot of work done in minimal time. Unlike cardio, where you might spend an hour training, HIIT can usually be done in 20 to 30 minutes, warm-up and cool down included. It does what it says on the tin: involves working out at a high intensity for a short duration, followed by a rest or low-intensity activity to let your heart rate drop back down.

4. Equipment for HIIT Workouts

4.1. Common Equipment Used in HIIT

4.2. Benefits of Using Equipment

5. 6 Best HIIT Exercises

5.1. Exercise 1: Burpees

5.2. Exercise 2: Mountain Climbers

5.3. Exercise 3: Jump Squats

5.4. Exercise 4: High Knees

5.5. Exercise 5: Plank Jacks

5.6. Exercise 6: Lateral Bounds

6. HIIT Workouts Without Equipment

Shedding fat and boosting cardiovascular health and endurance are all benefits of high-intensity interval training (HIIT). If you desire simpler bodyweight exercises that don't require any additional equipment, we've presented six different forms of HIIT exercise for you to try. Try each of these no-equipment niche movement intensifiers. For absolute newcomers, note the difficulty of each workout and work incrementally. Personal preferences can be a little subjective. If you're interested, take notes on how your body feels during each exercise. HIIT communicates and introduces diverse physical fitness avenues. In general, as a general rule of thumb, each HIIT should be followed by a short cool-down or mobility workout. Unwanted stress is reduced in this manner. To make things even more enjoyable, we've included an easy foam rolling cool-down for you to try!

If you're in a situation where you don't have the equipment you need for your workout, it doesn't necessarily mean that you can't get a great workout in. In fact, by executing bodyweight-based workouts and implementing movement quality, you can not only continue to make progress — but you can also become a better exerciser overall. Bodyweight exercises and the "Tabata" protocol (20 seconds of intense work followed by 10 seconds of rest repeated eight times) are generally repeatable workouts. Alternatively, hill sprints and high knees make a good workout. Because you can't sprint with maximal velocity for minutes on end, these short-burst activities provide an opportunity to rest. In normal weather, they alternate as a form of workout that causes metabolic disruption on the muscle level. Being able to create a serious burn is important. Much more than many of the "squat 500 times" protocols, shorter-range conditioning for physical and mental agility is essential. CustomButton HIIT: are unique explosive bursts — like jumping exercises or explosive sprints — instead of one-size-fits-all upper-body/lower-body exercise rep ranges (like kettlebell 15 three times) for a full-body workout that revolves around a single exercise for the upround phase. One rest is like a Tabata. Widening the lower-body repertoire is the focus of the first two rounds, with a series of upper-body explosive exercises following. If done properly, this tempo is almost guaranteed to maintain white-hot muscle adaptation. HIIT can be included all over the body!

Bodyweight HIIT workout: A combination of burpees, mountain climbers, tuck jumps, high knees, and squat jumps, this HIIT workout increases the heart rate and builds strength. Tabata: The Tabata protocol is an effective way to engage in high-intensity interval training. This four-minute routine consists of 20-second bouts of hard work, followed by a 10-second rest period, and it can be completed with or without equipment. Hill sprints: Something as simple as sprinting up a hill can be an effective form of high-intensity interval training without the need for equipment. High knees: Performing high knees, in place or while moving forward, in quick succession. Judo push-up: A bodyweight exercise that targets the chest, shoulders, triceps, and core. 1010-For-10 HIIT: This bodyweight circuit features 10 exercises done for 10 reps for 10 rounds. It alternates between lower-body moves and upper-body moves for efficiency and can be done almost anywhere at any time. The one downside of this workout is that the continuous lower-body activation may not be ideal for some exercises since they can begin building fatigue that limits performance in subsequent moves. With 120 seconds of rest between rounds, the 1010 For 10 HIIT workout can be performed in 30-40 minutes. The exercises in this workout include squats, push-ups, glute bridges, burpees, bicep curls, jumping jacks, tricep dips, lunges, crunches, and bicycle crunches.

6.1. Bodyweight Circuit Routine

Following is a simple beginner workout: Perform 50 each of: - Jumping jacks - Bodyweight squats - Mount climbers - Plank jacks - Walking lunges - Step ups on a bench or step - Pike push-ups - Leg lifts and climbers on back - Burpees

No doubt you can see this term in the magazine or online. The real question is why does it work? There is a simple explanation of the term HIIT, basically all you are doing is power jumping with bodyweight, max effort for 30 sec, then take 15-20 sec of rest. Because of all these main reasons it is placed number 1. To further explain, the reason why deduction docsn't work with these all-out type of exercises is during the off times, you can still push it with a very low or no impact form, and work those in-between sets.

When it comes to high-intensity interval training (HIIT), the common denominator is that you are either alternating between a period of work and a period of rest of the same exercise or alternating between two exercises. This article is going to cover just that with workouts for those people who don't want to go to gyms or stick to fancy treadmills and bikes. Send your calories burning by bodyweight.

Option 1

6.2. Tabata Protocol

The Tabata Protocol is one of the most recognized forms of HIIT, requiring no equipment. Named after Japanese exercise physiologist Izumi Tabata himself, the idea of the protocol is to adopt a 2:1 work-to-rest ratio. The basic format is: 20 seconds of full intensity exercise, followed by 10 seconds of rest. These 30 seconds are completed 8 times to reach a 4-minute round of high-intensity work. There is no allowance for a warm-up in Tabata. Participants go straight into one of the protocol's exercises. Cooldowns are suggested after all four rounds have been completed. If an individual is exercising less frequently, such as just two to three times a week, Vo2 workouts of this nature should be considered. Tabata is frequently referred to as High-Intensity Training (Effort Level) (HITEL). Although this is an appropriate use of the term, we will differentiate Tabata as HIIT after it is completed.

Sports and HIIT training cannot be separated; thus, the intensity of training systems has introduced a speed bag in the sporting world as High-Intensity Interval Training (HIIT). As the name implies, HIIT workouts consist of short and intense bursts of exercises, combined with active recovery, to keep the heart rate up and help burn more fat than moderate-intensity workouts. HIIT workouts have two main types: those that use equipment and those that do not use equipment (also called non-equipment HIIT workouts). The following list details 6 of the best HIIT exercises, both with and without equipment, to get you started with HIIT.

7. Creating Your Own HIIT Workout Routine

Warm-up and cool-down: Warm up your glutes, quads, hamstrings, calves, and feet using dynamic stretching exercises or similar movements. You can also increase your range of motion or start slowly with an exercise that mimics the intended activity. After completing a warm-up, begin a basic movement of a chosen exercise at a slower pace. Increase the intensity as you reach your target exercise pace. After completing this portion of the workout, perform static stretching exercises, such as hamstring, calf, hip, tricep, and shoulder stretches. Using a foam roller on a muscle for 30-60 seconds will help reduce muscle tension and improve flexibility. Cool down by walking or pedaling for three to five minutes before entering this phase and extending the post-workout static stretching workout routine.

The exercise list: Once you understand the purpose of your workout, choose what type of exercise you want to do. Here's a list of the best HIIT exercises we've covered so far. Choose from these exercises based on your goals, available space, or current level of resistance. Include this list into your workout plan, including at least one push, pull, leg, cardio, and core workout.

Setting goals: What do you want to accomplish with a HIIT workout routine? Choose an exercise that will help you meet these objectives. Because the format is "high intensity" and "interval training," HIIT is an excellent way to incorporate strength training and cardio into one workout. Plan to alternate between these two types of exercise for maximum results. If your primary interests are endurance improvements and interval work, you can adapt HIIT within these sports.

7.1. Setting Goals and Objectives

The five principles of your HIIT training session are: the work portion, the rest portion, the intensity, your work-to-rest ratio, and the sequence of exercises. Before you start, do a quick warm-up session to get your muscles moving. You can walk, jump, or jog in place for about 60 seconds. You can also warm up by stretching your core and legs before you begin. If you're doing a bodyweight HIIT workout, no equipment is needed. Wall sit is a great way to strengthen your legs. Place your back against a wall and then lower your body until your thighs are parallel to the ground. Hold the position for 45 seconds, engaging your core the entire time. Squat up and down for 45 seconds, then rest for 15 seconds. A push-up to side plank is a great upper-body exercise. For 45 seconds, do as many as you can. Once again, rest for 15 seconds. Place your hands on the ground, shoulder-width apart. That's all there is to it.

So, the big question here is what are your goals? No, none of that "I just want to look good" mumbo-jumbo. If you have clear and achievable fitness objectives, you're far more likely to meet them. A pound of fat equals 3500 calories. To lose a pound of fat within a week, you'll need to use 500 calories more than you consume every day. Most HIIT workouts range from about 15 to 30 minutes. Do this about three times a week, and you can lose about 0.5 to 1 pound of body fat per week. Resistance training is great for adding muscle, but it shouldn't be your only activity. Get at least 150 minutes of moderate cardio or 75 minutes of intense cardio each week. With vigorous activity, you should add muscle-strengthening activities at least twice per week. Make sure you're working out your major muscle groups: core, legs, arms, shoulders, chest, and back.

7.2. Choosing Exercises and Intervals

After a decision about the variety of exercises, the intervals will be chosen. Although it is rather typical that exercise selection affects the repetition times and brings a longer interval with a running machine, and breath-refreshing exercises for the second, the opposite approach can be beneficial, shifting the focus once again from the absolute physical intensity towards an integrative approach also with psychological reactions. Another option is to consider integration and the specificity of the intervals based on the effect they have on the energy system and choose accordingly. So, after all the choices, it is likely that a final choice can be made for certain situations without any reference to a golden rule, but taking individual and/or athletes' preferences into consideration with a focus on creativity and pleasure.

HIIT is an effective way of exercising, but it has to be personalized to be performed safely and effectively. To make a decision about the exercises and their variety, it is important to focus on the reason for performing HIIT training in the first place. HIIT should be considered with the main goal to improve physical fitness (and not the secondary goal to lose weight or improve health-related parameters, although they can be positively affected as well). It has to be emphasized that HIIT training should be intentionally performed to enhance physical condition. Thereby, exercises chosen to train the aerobic and anaerobic system should be used. Concerning the intensity, a classification of different zones like in "traditional" cardiorespiratory training can be used, focusing on the same road of developing a personal HIIT routine.

7.2. Choosing Exercises and Intervals

7.3. Warm-Up and Cool Down

After training, the cooling down period, during which the activity gradually decreases in intensity and works your implementing recovery, reduces the potential that you will 'hobble the session back' because you went too hard, as well as limiting the chances of feeling so gosh-darned painful in the day or two after training that you are forced to miss your next session or put your workout on hold. Essentially, the objective of a playing inactivity that encourages blood and oxygen flow to miss and fuel your muscles, as well as realign your temperature and slow your heart rate down in a controlled manner.

Warmed up fully, the cardiovascular system will be able to move blood effectively and efficiently throughout the body, and your joints and muscles will work more gracefully and function better, all of which adds to a better workout. Not just that, research has, in fact, demonstrated that knee and ankle power, strength, and Durnin concluded that not warming up gorgeously could increase athletic potential and reduce the risk for decisively injury. A study published by the Blackwell Institute showed that as a result of not warming up, athletes would have scored a goal in soccer 14% of the time. That is right; there is very real science to back the take that not warming up could even imperially affect your performance at the gym, as well as being beneficial in-class and to general athletes. Warming up will help your performance at work, within your show or Saceutical, or help you do better at home with your family.

Importance of the Warm-up and the Cool Down

8. Conclusion and Final Tips

In conclusion, it's important to know your limits and be aware of your current fitness level. Speak to your personal trainer before adding new workouts to your routine - it is important that they are tailored to you. Especially as the Fitness Manager at No1 Fitness, it is the sort of thing I'd like you to speak to one of the fitness managers about. If at any time during a workout you're feeling any discomfort, please stop and contact a fitness professional. Our team of personal trainers at No1 Fitness would be happy to help you with correct form, building a nutritional plan, ensuring your workouts are effective and injury-free, as well as being there to support, motivate, and encourage you to achieve your goals.

- HIIT workouts should last no longer than 30 minutes. - These workouts are based on extremely high- and low-intensity intervals that help the body to burn fat. - You can do HIIT either at a gym or do body-weight workouts at home. - Warm-up and cool-down are very important. - Be aware that you might need a recovery system, like foam rolling. - Nutrition is key, regarding both pre- and post-workout nutrition.

What HIIT has going for it is that it has been shown to be three times more effective at burning fat over traditional or steady-state cardio. This is because it boosts your metabolism, meaning you'll continue to burn fat even after you've ended training. Now that we have done a deep dive into HIIT, let us now take stock of all the key takeaways:

Incorporating High-Intensity Interval Training (HIIT) into Your Fitness Routine

1. Introduction to HIIT

Incorporating HIIT into your fitness routine is imperative for a well-rounded workout! It provides just as good if not better results than longer workouts, offers greater strength improvements, helps burn fat more efficiently by burning more fat throughout the day, allows you more freedom in exercise choices and variety, and gives you more free time. HIIT is best used to bust through plateaus in aerobic exercise performance and/or strength improvements and change up exercise routines for variety. Always remember to get your doctor's permission to do HIIT workouts, as they can be extreme!

The routine of HIIT varies from person to person, but in general, a HIIT workout consists of intense exercise for 30 seconds to 4 minutes, followed by rest or low-intensity exercise that lasts at least that long. A 2:1 rest-to-work ratio is generally recommended, and the average routine lasts 30 minutes - warmup and cool-down included.

In recent years, researchers and dieters have been raving about the benefits of high-intensity interval training (HIIT). The reason for this lies in its unique approach to exercising: HIIT essentially pairs bouts of very hard exercise with smaller bouts of lower-intensity exercise. Research shows that this method of training burns more fat and builds more muscle than traditional long cardio workouts. In fact, HIIT is so beneficial that fitness experts predict it will be the top fitness trend of 2022.

2. Benefits of HIIT

The most obvious attraction to HIIT workouts may be the speed in which you can burn calories relative to consistent paced workouts. Intensity forces your body to work harder and uses up more stored energy but is also often not as easy to recover from. However, the benefits can include improving cardiovascular health – which corresponds with improved fitness and endurance. Regular HIIT training can also improve your blood pressure and heart rate, again contributing to improved overall heart health, reducing the risk of more serious health concerns. Cholesterol and blood sugar are also positively affected, with fat utilization often improving. While the intensity does, in itself, promote calorie burning, the workout's afterburn effect means that you will continue to expend energy after the session as your body works hard to replenish any lost glycogen. This is also known as EPOC (Excess Post-Exercise Oxygen Consumption). Overall, due to the impressive payoff for an intense but short amount of effort, far less time is required to get a good workout completed.

While there are a plethora of different training styles and programs out there, one of the most popular methods right now is High Intensity Interval Training – or HIIT. Not only does it enable you to burn a lot of calories more quickly, but there are some awesome health benefits associated with HIIT too. HIIT workouts generally focus on increasing your heart rate through quick, intense spurts of physical activity for a brief period, followed by a short rest period.

The process is then repeated as a full set, with multiple sets planned per workout. This whole process can be completed in 20-30 minutes, with short workouts tailored for people who are short of time.

3. Getting Started with HIIT

First things first, set a goal you can actually reach. Remember how important it is to discuss your level of comfort and areas of concern with your physician. You have to stay consistent with whatever activities you choose. The whole point of HIIT is to keep your heart rate up with short bursts of brisk or intense movements. Think of exercises you are comfortable with and do not require specialized equipment. A proper warm-up and cool down are also essential to your physical safety. Overall, the sequence of warm-up, high-intensity movement, recovery movement, and cool down should last between 30 minutes and 1 hour. Remember to start your cool down 5-10 minutes before you wrap up the activities. This segment should include a brief 'mega' stretch of some kind. Just be sure to give your heart a heads up that its work is almost finished. Design a workout for variety. Exercise more than 12 minutes at 70% max and commit to at least 20 minutes of your favorite style of HIIT three or more days every week. This style aligns with most every type of lifestyle. All styles of interval training involve varying intensities of running, biking, walking, general bodyweight or a combination of these activities through some kind of challenge. Short sprints, high knees, fast feet, and helping hands can be combined with slower, resting activities just like longer, slower vintages of exercise with this new insight. HIIT: a tool for your fitness.

3.1. Setting Realistic Goals

The motivations to begin a fitness routine should all be timebound, approachable, and evidence that motivation comes from within. This will be different for each client. If this motivation doesn't materialize, the client is not likely to persist with a HIIT lifestyle. As a practitioner, we can support, lead, guide, relate, and understand each client's motivation from the outset.

First and foremost, the fitness enthusiast's ambition for the HIIT must be to build an intrinsic passion for exercise. A focus on outward battle will never defeat the inward war. The commitment to HIIT requires lifelong dedication. It demands proper nutrition, ample sleep, and dedication to rooting out destructive habits of the past. The real rewards of this "fitness lifestyle" occur not on the body, but inside the body.

The fundamental importance of setting clear, concise, and realistic goals when beginning a HIIT regimen should not be underestimated. Goals that are too unrealistic can therefore lead to feelings of inferiority when they are not achieved. Part of the battle in achieving a successful fitness regimen extends to creating a sense of progress, a feat most easily achieved when persistent, myopic, and contextually appropriate goals are the pursuit. Because, the genuineness of HIIT is to bear witness to long-term and evident changes. It sets its own pace on that silver platter of promised improvement. Outward appearance cannot be what drives the state forward. It delegitimizes the intrinsic factoring of progress and raw personal willpower. Many individuals struggle with motivation during the beginning stages of fitness. This is due to the lack of ease and personal performance of the movements and usage of the gym equipment. Therefore, it is important that the motivations to begin a fitness are realistic from the get-go.

3.1. Setting realistic goals

Incorporating high-intensity interval training (HIIT) into your fitness routine

3.2. Choosing the Right Exercises

Choose exercises you can perform. They may not be perfect at first, but they should be something you can do within the specified rep range and still keep good form. Know your intensities according to the goals of your workout. Intensity is a key factor in every workout. The level of intensity that you can produce is a factor that depends on your goals. If your workout has a goal to increase your strength, then the intensity should be high, up to 85% of your 1-rep max or even higher. If you should perform a workout on the other hand, with a goal to improve your endurance, then the intensity should be lower, like 30-40% of your 1-rep max. Know your aims of the workout. Similarly to the level of intensity, the specific aims determine not only what type of structure you are going to follow but also the intensity that is appropriate.

When selecting movements to perform in a high-intensity interval training (HIIT) workout, you should keep in mind all facets of fitness: cardiovascular conditioning, strength, and power. More specifically, HIIT workouts should consist of multi-joint movements that engage both the upper and lower body, activated on both the concentric and eccentric portions of every repetition. Beyond that, the individual fitness level of the athlete and their specific training goals should be taken into consideration.

3.3. Creating a HIIT Workout Plan

The most important thing you'll need to decide when planning your HIIT workouts is what kind of exercises you're planning on doing. Many people choose only bodyweight exercises like burpees, mountain climbers, push-ups, etc. Others opt (or also include) weighted exercises like kettlebell swings, box jumps or weighted squats. Unlike traditional cardio exercises where you may do the same movement at the same intensity for an extended period of time, HIIT exercises should vary. Not only does this minimize burnout by preventing overuse of the same muscle group, but it also encourages a more balanced application of strength and endurance. Finally, it's lineup time! In addition to your various exercises, you should also plan your rest periods between intervals. The duration of your rest is ultimately up to you, but more importantly when considering this factor, is consistency. If you're just beginning and need to rest for 45 seconds between intervals, try to keep that duration consistent across your entire workout. The single day you finally manage to rest for 30 seconds instead of 45 is the exact day you'll need to stop early. Lastly, keep increasing the difficulty every two weeks or so to make HIIT a sustainable and effective part of your routine.

One of the beautiful things about HIIT is how easy it is to tailor a workout to your specific interests, but perhaps the most common questions from those new to HIIT is how long and hard each 'working' interval should be. The answer, as always, is that it depends! It depends on your skill level, as well as lifestyle factors. For example, three 30-second sprints might be perfect for someone who typically only works from the couch to the refrigerator, but of course, you'll want to advance to longer intervals if you're more athletic.

4. Progressing in HIIT

More advanced exercises. Once you've established variations of high knees, burpees, tuck jumps, and mountain climbers, you can search for more advanced exercises to include in your workout, such as plyometric pushups and broad jumps. Once you have a firm grasp on one style of HIIT, regressing back to moderate intensity steady-state cardio and building up again can also help to keep your body guessing and prevent hitting a training plateau. This may mean cycling several sprints instead of propping up on a bike seat during a flat-out RPM workout, or skipping on the spot rather than completing a 100m sprint. Advanced progressions can include active recovery sessions between intervals (either steady-state moderate intensity endurance or less intense/intimidating versions of the high-intensity movements).

Increase intensity gradually. To see results and avoid injury, it's important to overload your body. Gradually increase the number of intervals or duration of work. If you're doing 20 seconds of work, start by upping it to 25 seconds four weeks into your routine, then 30 seconds six weeks in. This gradual increase can be applied to both time and effort, with newbies starting off with a 1:2 intensity ratio of work to recovery, while intermediates can up their weights and reduce recovery to a 1:1 ratio. Allowing 0-90 seconds of recovery between sets is usually a sweet spot for those beginning their HIIT journey, while 0-60 seconds is considered adequate for intermediates.

We progressively overload in weights, so it makes sense to change up HIIT every 4-8 weeks. Once you are comfortable with one type of exercise, begin upping the intensity of your workout before integrating more advanced exercises into your routine.

4.1. Increasing Intensity

Once you have a substantial base and routinely incorporate a hefty portion of sprints into your routine, that's when we switch to HIIT. Here is where the "ass-kicker" HIIT workouts begin. While moderate-intensity workouts like tempo runs can help you increase your running pace and stamina, HIIT takes it a notch higher, as it taxes your body by triggering high-intensity workouts in short bursts. Keep in mind that races, speed workouts, long days, and other higher impact workouts can increase the likelihood of overload and injury.

The beauty of HIIT workouts is that they can evolve with you. If you're starting out but making headway, every day is a perfect time to intensify them. In this phase, focus on running faster and longer. Before transitioning to the "ass-kicker" workouts that launch you into a bout of sprint training, you need to ensure that you have a baseline of endurance and strength pertinent to completing HIIT sessions (not recommended for beginners). Even though you may progress to "ass-kicker" HIIT workouts, it's still prudent to perform sprints closer to your 5k and 2-mile pace due to the high likelihood of hamstring pull or ACL tear. Focus on building your VO2 max with a mixture of easy runs, tempo runs, and threshold runs, so your body can physically handle the increase in intensity without being at a greater injury risk.

4.2. Incorporating Advanced Exercises

Incorporate the kind of workout that works for you. Maybe you're OK with running during your HIIT workouts, but you'd prefer to climb on the bike when you're not in the gym. Great! Why not do your interval work in a way that you're comfortable with and that you're looking forward to? Our goal is to find exercises and combinations that you find most beneficial. Combinations of high-resistance exercises, such as weightlifting, for instance, are quite effective as well. A beginner's workout is one that you're comfortable working out in. If 8 to 12 reps are easy for you, add a cycle of weighted squats and include that in your HIIT routine. Using advanced exercises in your HIIT routine, like the deadlift, is something you can work toward if you go beyond a beginner fitness level. Listen to your body. Go to the gym and never overexert your body and set records for reps or weight lifts too soon. Always listen to your body, and be careful.

These basic forms of high-intensity interval training should give you a great foundation for putting what you've learned into practice. HIIT is really something you can tailor specifically to your training depending on what your fitness goals are. For instance, if you're a runner or a cyclist, you may want to incorporate longer efforts on the lower end of the HIIT spectrum, making them more like "tempo" efforts. It takes a bit of experimentation to make it work for you, but once you find the right mix, you'll know it. If you're less experienced in creating your own workouts, don't hesitate to seek help from a trainer. HIIT can be a great way to incorporate advanced exercises into your program, but like everything else, be sure not to include it all the time.

4.2. Incorporating Advanced Exercises

5. Consistency in HIIT

There's a very real physiological mechanism behind these plateaus. In short, your body hasn't completely adapted to your new routine, lessening the stress and thus demand on your body. And when your body isn't challenged as much, you'll see less pronounced results. But not all plateaus are solely physiologically based. You might face other "internal" roadblocks – like stress, scheduling, or just plain old fatigue. Internal factors can change things, but external factors might give you a new perspective on getting back on the HIIT track.

Regardless of your goals, one crucial component of any HIIT workout is the ability to get you sweating. In fact, studies show that HIIT workouts can help you break a sweat and improve overall blood circulation more effectively than moderate-intensity workouts.

Get your heart pumping. Regardless of the type of workout you pick, pay attention to what happens once you dial the intensity up. Your heart begins to work harder, sending oxygen and nutrient-rich blood to your hard-working muscles, bones, and organs. That's because your body is working overtime to support optimal brain function while feeding your hungry muscles with the fuel they need to keep up.

Perhaps most importantly, incorporating HIIT into your routine means consistency. Researchers have found that a total-body HIIT workout built around 60-second intervals can give you the most bang for your buck. If you're just starting out, aim to do a HIIT workout twice a week, gradually building up to four times per week.

5.1. Establishing a Routine

On the practical side of how to make this happen, prioritize workouts in the morning as much as possible. Planning a strength and conditioning class, whole-body workout, or another workout session in the mornings is a good way to ensure that you do not bail on it later due to exhaustion or work-related stresses. Morning workouts also help to facilitate maximum fat and calorie burn at the start of the day, which helps to prepare you for the most beneficial diet-related decisions. For ease of life and interest in workouts, it is best to try to hit a few different kinds of exercise per season, or at least per year. Keep track of your interests and the activities that you enjoy the most, because those are the activities that will be most likely to stick with you for a lifetime.

To get the most out of a high-intensity interval training (HIIT) routine, the most important thing that you can do is to make it a rule to use working out as part of a routine. Incorporating exercise into the routine in this way allows for the highest likelihood that you will be able to keep up regular exercise — which is effectively the 'secret' to gaining any kind of benefit from a full-body workout. Schedule your workouts. Mark them on your calendar as though they are an official appointment. The larger that you can make exercise a part of your routine, the more consistent you will become, and the more compelling your results in the future.

5.2. Overcoming Plateaus

When following an exercise program, self-motivation plays a major role in progressing. Psychological approaches will help maintain motivation, despite tough times or perceived lack of results early in the program. The two most important manners from a psychological perspective about overcoming a plateau are to appreciate the small strides of accomplishment and to maintain motivation. Mistakenly, people tend to have high expectations when they first begin an exercise or weight loss program. When greater and faster advances are not achieved as quickly as an exerciser desires, he or she loses interest and "throws in the towel." Especially when beginning a new routine, it is important for trainers to point out even little achievements - being able to perform an exercise (greater balance, agility, or range of motion), being able to incorporate some kind of progression on a machine. Let them know their bones are getting denser and their hearts are getting stronger. Many people give up and stop working out because they get discouraged after not losing 20 pounds or dropping three dress sizes in a month. Even eliminating just 3 pounds is an extremely good start that is helping to achieve a healthier lifestyle! Exercise is about being a change for life and becoming stronger and leaner. Documentary studies and some people make statements to thank the muscle builders because even if they have lost the extra weight, they have been supported by a stronger body and renewed self-esteem.

Maintain motivation

Implementing variety into HIIT is another strategy to turn things around. Variety has been reported to combat repetitive strenuous efforts that can impinge on an individual's ability to physically and mentally continue to advance. While the principle formula for HIIT training may be set by the interval duration, rest duration, and the number of repetitions or total time, slight fluctuations in the amount of time according to how an exerciser may "feel" can be manipulated (i.e., level of fatigue versus an overexerted state) to elicit more adaptations. For instance, if an exerciser has the tolerance and is no longer working hard at 1 to 2 minutes, he or she may decrease the rest time to 15 seconds or reduce it to 1-minute all-outs with 3 to 4 minutes of rest. Other ways to introduce variety include training in the morning one day or the evening the next, and doing long HIIT one week and short HIIT the next. HIIT class participants may find that varying music, teaching style, or workouts as a means of providing variety can help motivate participants. Listening to music that participants do not like, in contrast, will dim the exerciser's attitude. Including a strong support system is the final strategy of the psychologist.

Whether it's in strength, speed, endurance, or overall progress, the potential to experience a plateau period, especially for new or inexperienced exercisers, can be frustrating and derail someone from wanting to continue in a program. Several strategies, however, can be used to continuously advance in HIIT. The first two strategies adjust the workout variables of HIIT training. Variables such as time, intensity (using a different exercise that works the same muscle groups at the same time and in the same way), and work-to-rest ratios can be manipulated to elicit improvements when the participant appears to be at a standstill or begins regressing.

6. Conclusion and Final Tips

In conclusion, I hope that for those of you who have made it to the end of this paper have garnered, at the very least, an improved understanding of HIIT. My hope is that if you are a mandated reader, for any reason pertaining to the field of health and fitness, you feel as though you have gained an adequate amount of knowledge and insight into the wonderful world of high-intensity training to augment your pre-existing knowledge base. With the novel implementation of HIIT education, there were certainly many objectives in mind. The most critical of these three objectives – from my perspective – are the following: to provide a comprehensive and thorough description and analysis of the very concept of HIIT, to unpack the precise science that provides the merit for the training style, and to provide readers with various methods with which they might explore and develop as part of their repertoire. For the trainers, this chapter was developed especially to provide some insight into activities or methods that may assist with training, development or management. In the same fashion, I aimed to deliver a comprehensive, evidence-based understanding and overview of HIIT. I wanted to provide a clear, scientific insight into the benefits – stress and otherwise – of HIIT so that people could use this information in their practice or apply it to their training or life. I aspire that this research and the various aspects of this paper undergo exploration and development and critique. Please don't hesitate to let me know if you have any thoughts.

In conclusion, it is vital to understand high-intensity interval training (HIIT) for various reasons. Firstly, it is a very effective workout style that you can add or incorporate into your current routine to continue progressing. Secondly, if you are time-poor, its efficacy can ensure your fitness does not suffer. My three biggest tips for someone looking to start incorporating HIIT are as follows: firstly, select a HIIT style that appeals to you such as LISS HIIT if you enjoy walking, Tabata if you are not particularly fond of cardio, and progressive if you have programmed workouts. Find an interval that challenges you, and lastly, listen to your body. HIIT doesn't suit or appeal to everyone, and that is okay. Just because it is a current trend doesn't mean it is the only way to burn calories or lose a centimeter off your waistline.